T0205773

Craniomandibular Dysfunction in Violinists

Riema Abdunnur

Craniomandibular Dysfunction in Violinists

A Literature Review

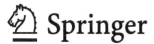

Riema Abdunnur
Medical University of Innsbruck
Innsbruck, Austria

Dissertation, Medical University of Innsbruck, 2017

Additional material to this book can be downloaded from http://extras.springer.com.

ISBN 978-3-658-24147-6   ISBN 978-3-658-24148-3   (eBook)
https://doi.org/10.1007/978-3-658-24148-3

Library of Congress Control Number: 2018960352

This Springer imprint is published by the registered company Springer Fachmedien Wiesbaden GmbH
part of Springer Nature
The registered company address is: Abraham-Lincoln-Str. 46, 65189 Wiesbaden, Germany

Acknowledgement

This work would not have been possible without the support of many people. My heartfelt gratitude goes to Professor Dr. Dr. Ingrid Grunert, my main supervisor, for her excellent scientific guidance and efforts to make this work a reality. My sincere appreciation also goes to Professor Dr. Rudolf Bratschko, my co-supervisor, for his scientific input. Many special thanks go to DT. Manfred Läkamp, for his guidance and great encouragement.

Special gratitude goes also to the wonderful orchestral musician Martina Overlöper, and to the syrian biologist M.Sc. Hadeel Shammas, who both offered me great support.

Many thanks go yet to my colleagues in the post gradual master study program "Craniomandibular and Musculoskeletal Medicine – CMM" who kept helping and encouraging me to find my new way here in Germany, after leaving Syria, my first and beloved homeland.

My wonderful husband and children were been a strong source of encouragement and understanding all the time. They endured this long process with me, always offering support and love. Without you I wouldn't have been able to reach anything of this.

Thank you all.

Riema Abdunnur

Table of Content

List of Figures

List of Abbreviations

AAOP	American Academy of Orofacial Pain
CMD	Craniomandibular dysfunction
CMS	Craniomandibular system
EMG / sEMG	Electromyography / surface Electromyography
IRT	Infrared thermal imaging
MMS	Musculoskeletal system
MPA	Music performance anxiety
MPS	Myofascial pain syndrome
MTrPs	Myofascial trigger points
NAREMG	Normalized average rectified electromyography
OPG	Orthopantomogram
PRMDs	Playing-related musculoskeletal disorders
RCD/TMD	Research diagnostic criteria/Temporo mandibular disorders
SCM	Sternocleidomastoid muscle
TMD	Temporomandibular dysfunction (disorder)
TMJ	Temporomandibular joint
TrPs	Trigger Points

Zusammenfassung

Hintergrund und Ziele

Musiker, die Geige spielen, sind anfällig für bestimmte Arten von orofazialen Problemen und prädisponiert, Craniomandibuläre Dysfunktionen (CMD) zu entwickeln. Diese These gibt einen Einblick auf Publikationen, die sich auf Geigern konzentrieren, vor allem auf die, die an einer CMD leiden. Damit erzielt sie ein besseres Verständnis für die einzigartigen Arbeitsbedingungen von Geigern und die Verbesserung der diagnostischen und therapeutischen Ergebnisse bei praktizierenden Zahnärzten. Darüber hinaus ist das Ziel der Analyse der Publikationen zu ermitteln, was genau bei den Geigern in Bezug auf CMD bisher recherchiert wurde und wie weit die manuelle Medizin darin eingeschlossen war.

Materialen und Methoden

Eine Literatursuche der PubMed Datenbank der National Library of Medicine wurde in englischer und deutscher Sprache ohne zeitliche Einschränkungen durchgeführt. Schlüsselwörter waren (craniomandibular disorder) AND (violin). Diese Suche ergab zwölf Artikel, von denen acht in diesem Review enthalten sind. Ähnliche Studien und deren Referenzen wurden nach weiteren Artikeln gesucht. Zudem wurden in deutscher Sprache veröffentlichten Büchern mit musikspezifischen Krankheiten nach relevanten Informationen recherchiert.

Ergebnisse

Die endgültige Anzahl der eingeschlossenen Studien waren zehn Artikel, von denen sieben nach dem PICO-Prozess analysiert wurden, während drei Fall-Kontrollen nur zusammengefasst wurden.

Diskussion und Schlussfolgerung

Diese These schafft einen Überblick über die Literatur in Bezug auf CMD bei Geigern und analysiert eine Reihe von Studien. Viele analysierten Studien deuten auf eine mögliche Assoziation zwischen CMD und das Spielen der Geige. Im Allgemeinen werden in der Zukunft mehr Forschungen empfohlen, die dieses Thema in Erwägung ziehen, vor allem jene, die die nach den biomechanischen Effekten des Geigenspielens an CMD leidenden Geigern recherchieren, und solche, die diese Patienten via kooperierenden Konzepten zwischen Zahnmedizin und manueller Medizin diagnostizieren und behandeln.

Abstract

Background and Aims

Musicians who play Violin are prone to particular types of orofacial problems and are predisposed to develop Craniomandibular Dysfunction (CMD). This paper gives insight into publications focussing on performing violinists, particularly on those suffering from CMD, subsequently providing a better understanding to the unique work conditions of violinists, and enhancing diagnosis and therapeutic results by practitioner dentists. Moreover, the analysis of the included papers aims to reveal what exactly was studied in violinists regarding to CMD, and how far manual medicine was included there.

Materials and Methods

A literature search of The National Library of Medicine's PubMed database was conducted in English and German without time restrictions. The key words used were (craniomandibular disorder) AND (violin). This search yielded twelve articles, eight of which are included in this review. Similar papres and references of all articles were searched for other articles to be selected. In addition, books that were published in German language with music-specific diseases were also searched for relevant information.

Results

The final number of included studies that met the inclusion criteria was ten articles, seven of which were analysed according to the "PICO process" (Population, Intervention, Control, Outcome); whereas three case reports were only summarised.

Discussion and Conclusion

This thesis reveals an overview of the literature in terms of CMD in violinists and analyses a number of papers. Many analysed papers suggest a possible association between CMD and playing the violin. In general, more researches considering this topic are recommended in the future, especially those handling biomechanical effects of the violin on players suffering from CMD, and those diagnosing and treating such patients via cooperating concepts between dentistry and manual medicine.

1 Introduction

In creating and performing music, musicians can experience health problems from the high physical and psychological demands of their profession [1]. The expert musician demonstrates spatial and temporal accuracy and coordination equivalent to that of Olympic athletes [2]. Ten thousand hours of accumulated practice over approximately ten years is necessary to achieve elite levels of performance [3]. This method is not foolproof for producing individuals capable of performing their motor skills in safest, most efficient manner possible. So musicians and athletes share another less desirable characteristic: developing performance-related injuries [4].

Musculoskeletal complaints are one of the main medical problems among musicians [5-7]. Excessive muscle tension is viewed as a significant causal factor in musicians' injuries [8]. Muscle tension can be incurred as a result of the postures required to support an instrument, in addition to the physical activities needed for performance. In particular, the violin and viola are potentially problematic because they are totally supported by body of the player [9]. Fine motor motions have to be performed with a spatial precision of fractions of millimeters and with a temporal accuracy of milliseconds mostly in coordination with other musicians, so that muscles, nerves and joints are often brought to the limit of their physiological performance. It is therefore not surprising that such a high-performance system is more susceptible to disturbances [10].

Musculoskeletal disorders related to playing an instrument are painful, chronic and disabling conditions which are prevalent among classical musicians. Zaza defined these Playing-related musculoskeletal disorders (PRMDs) as personal and chronic health problems that affect the whole person, physically, emotionally, occupationally, socially and financially [1]. These can threaten the identity of professional musicians, so that some of them will stop playing their instrument due to these complaints [11].

Real interest in the health and well-being of musicians by medical practitioners, researchers and music professionals was developed since the 1980s [12]. Many of them were highly interested in health complaints in Violinists and were analyzing the effect of playing the Violin on developing Craniomandibular dysfunction CMD (also called Temporomandibular dysfunction TMD); an important form of PRMDs. The American Academy of Orofacial Pain (AAOP) defined TMD as a collective term embracing a number of clinical problems that involve the

© Springer Fachmedien Wiesbaden GmbH, part of Springer Nature 2019
R. Abdunnur, *Craniomandibular Dysfunction in Violinists*,
https://doi.org/10.1007/978-3-658-24148-3_1

masticatory musculature, temporomandibular joint (TMJ) and associated structures, or both [13].

TMD is a common disease, but the symptoms and problems could be manifested differently in each individual [14-16]. It also occurs more frequently in women than in men [17,18].

According to Steinmetz et al., causes of CMD could be classified in 3 categories: 1. Occlusiogenic, as seen in malocclusions 2. Myogenic, by parafunctions such as bruxism or postural disturbances or muscular imbalances 3. Arthrogenic, due to internal derangement or arthritis of the temporomandibular joint [10]. According to Graber, stress (with its pronounced effect on the muscular system) as well as psycho-emotional aspects, are also a significant reinforcing factor [19-23]. Thus, psyche has to be considered as an indispensable factor in the pathogenesis of CMD.

In the existing literature, it has been reported that many instruments, such as bowed strings, flute, guitar, and trombone, require the player to work constantly in an asymmetric playing posture [24-27]. The instrument is held with one arm elevated, which demands a static muscle load to stabilize the shoulder blade and shoulder joint. With some instruments, players also have to rotate and bend the head and hold their lower back turned to one side, which may lead to unilateral, static muscle work [28].

The position of the head in relation to the trunk has not only influence on the cervical spine function, but also on the versatile functions of the movement apparatus of the chewing system [29]. Some postural abnormalities and symmetry disturbances outside of the stomatognathic area can be the cause of CMD [30].

Vice versa, Patients with pain in the cervical spine, the lumbar spine and the pelvic floor have usually also dysfunctions of the temporomandibular joints and the occlusion, which varies in their quality and quantity and are therefore often ignored [31].

Considering the previous mentioned facts, I've decided in this review to deal also with studies discussing the asymmetric muscular functions which violinists have to face while performing, not only in the head, but also in the neck and shoulder regions, aiming to give a comprehensive sight into their CMD-problem.

1.1 Prevalence

String players belong to the instrument group that is often affected by playing-related complaints [32]. Concerning playing-related musculoskeletal disorders (PRMDs), it could be shown that almost 86 % of musicians were affected by these disorders. Upper string players, in particular violinists, demonstrated the highest prevalence ratios for neck, left shoulder and left wrist pain as well as frequently experiencing pain in more than five pain regions [33,34]. Musicians with string instrument (as main instrument) had twice the incidence of cervical spine, right shoulder and left elbow/forearm disorders compared to musicians who had piano as the main instrument [35]. Other studies have considered string instruments as the main risk music instruments [36,37]. The largest published study ever undertaken involving professional orchestra musicians surveyed a population of 4,025 musicians from 48 orchestras in the United States in 1986, in which players whose playing requires both repetitive actions and static loading had the highest risk of PRMDs (66 % prevalence), with the neck and shoulder being the prime sites affected [38,39]. Other studies revealed that upper limb performance-related injuries or pain affect from 50 % to 88 % of professional violinists [1,40,41]. By combining location of PRMD, instrument, and gender, the researchers found that female violin players had a significantly higher percentage of severe problems in both shoulders and both sides of the neck [39].

Concerning the prevalence of TMD among musicians, one study revealed that the incidence of TMD symptoms for musicians is similar to that of the general population, but these symptoms are activated and accentuated when performing or practicing music [42]. Oppositely, other studies show that violinists report pain in the neck, masseter and temporalis muscles more frequently than the population norm (40 per cent compared with 14 per cent) [43]. These significantly higher prevalence of CMD found in musicians made some authors consider "professsional violin play" as a possible predispositional factor for the development of a CMD [44,45].

1.2 Signs and Symptoms

Symptoms of CMD are characterized as following [10]:

1) Pain in the TMJs or chewing muscles.

2) Mandibular dysfunction in form of restriction in mouth opening and/or laterotrusion (lateral deflection of the lower jaw) during mouth opening.

3) TMJ sounds (clicking or crepitation).

In addition, symptoms outside of the masticatory system could be seen such as headache, otalgia, dizziness, globular sensation, lumbago, inclined pelvis and variable leg length difference. These complaints are often the focus of CMD patients and many of them describe their temporomandibular joints subjectively as symptom free [46]. Therefore, the temporomandibular joint is often not diagnosed as a cause of such symptoms. Moreover, the low subjective need for treatment in some patients is due to the fact that their pain doesn't manifest in the region of the TMJ but in the shoulder-neck region or even in the lumbosacral region [10].

Violinists are prone to TMJ disorders, particularly pain in the region of the right TMJ, due to the pressure on the mandible of holding the instrument and the clenching of the masticatory muscles [47]. Violin playing tend to push the mandible to the right and possibly also forward; the tenderness in the right lateral pterygoid muscle might therefore be due to the tendency to try to resist the "pushing effect" of the violin through this muscular hyperactivity. Furthermore, violinists using no shoulder support or only a cushion need more muscular force to bring the chin and the left shoulder closer together when holding the instrument, resulting in painful mandibular movements while clinical examination [48].

A larger deviation of the mandible in violinists to the right of the midline on maximal mouth opening was found compared with that for non-musician controls. It has been considered that excessive and/or prolonged force applied to the left mandible in holding the instrument is the main cause of their problems [44,49,50].

A survey with dental examination of musicians was undertaken in 2008 identified nearly three times more signs and symptoms of bruxism in violinists and violists than in non-musician controls [51]. A correlation was also found between tinnitus/impaired hearing and hours practicing on the violin [35]. Other researchers found that violinists in general show modified clinical findings compared with non-violin-playing controls; less maximal mouth opening with more pain while opening, more TMJ sounds, more painful mandibular movements and more deviation, more palpatory tenderness in their masticatory muscles, and more parafunctional habits [44,45,52].

Increased muscular load in the muscles of mastication, the trapezius, and the sternocleidomastoid muscles during playing the violin which can possibly predispose to overuse syndromes [10]. An overuse or overload syndrome is a condition in which muscles, tendons and ligaments are loaded beyond their physiological capacity [53,54]. Moreover, long-term playing of the violin can create CMD, that's why professional musicians often complain of pain in the neck, arm or shoulder [55].

Musicians can also experience considerable levels of stress due to the high physical and psychological demands of their profession. It is well known that psyche and soma are strongly linked to each other. Selye divided the "stress syndrome", or the "general adaptation syndrome" as he preferred to name it, in three stages: 1. Alarm reaction. 2. Phase of resistance. 3. Phase of exhaustion [56]. Fears lead to muscle tension, and persistent painful muscle tension leads to anxiety. Psychosomatically induced pain is largely associated with neuromuscular hypertension, which can turn into a hypotonia in long-lasting chronic course [57].

Chronic muscular tension is the origin of psychosomatic pain [58]. The resulting pain intensifies the cramp, which in turn intensifies the pain. In the case of psychosomatic pain, such as are found in the CMD, the triggering psychological, somatic and social factors are not to be exactly separated from each other. These factors are rather interrelated [57].

A recent study dealing with anxiety in performing musicians showed that violinists who reported TMD symptoms, were significantly associated with high levels of MPA (Music Performance Anxiety), therefore it was suggested to address both psychological and physical factors simultaneously in musicians who do not improve with physical therapy only [59].

1.3 Etiology and Predisposing Factors

The exact cause of developing a CMD in musicians is often not easy to recognize [15,16,31,60-62], since clear guiding symptoms are usually lacking. So it often can't be exactly ascertained whether existing TMJ problems affect the playing of a high stringed instrument or whether these complaints are triggered or amplified by the instrumental play [63]. Many researchers have found that a greater unilateral or bilateral loss of posterior occlusal support is directly related to a reduced condylar gap in both joints [64,65]. The triggers leading to a decompensation of occlusal disturbances are of a varied nature. There are factors that increase dysfunction and/or muscle activity such as stress, further occlusive disorders, metabolic and hormonal factors (thyroid disorders, etc.), trauma and ascending function disturbances, such as Posture [57] (Figure 1.1).

Since the temporomandibular joint is connected to the spinal column by means of bony, muscular and ligamentous connections, any disturbance in the TMJ therefore will not remain isolated in the masticating apparatus, but will affect the postures of both; head and body. Conversely, CMD may occur due to disorders outside the craniomandibular system, and changes in head and body posture can have a direct effect on the position of the temporomandibular joints and the relationship between the cranial bones [66-72].

Figure 1.2 shows skeletal and muscular interrelationships in the craniomandibular system CMS and the musculoskeletal system MMS [57]. Stiesch-Scholz et al. could find a significant comorbidity between patients with internal derangement of the TMJ and dysfunctions of the cervical spine without subjective neck problems [73]. Disturbances in the TMJ area, occlusion or masticatory muscles could therefore be associated with dysfunctions or complex pain syndromes in other areas of the body: Floor of the mouth head joints, spine, hyoid bone, diaphragm, pelvis and even internal organs [10].

It is also evident that CMDs are frequently associated with pain and discomfort in the shoulder and the whole upper extremity and are presumed to contribute to an increased muscular load and activity in these regions, especially in the sterno-cleidomastoid and trapezius muscles that demonstrate increased resting activities in patients with CMD [74,75]. Additionally, parafunctional activities like clenching are also proven to increase resting muscle activity for the sternocleido-mastoid and trapezius muscles, as well as for trunk muscles: lumbar paravertebral and rectus abdominis muscles [76].

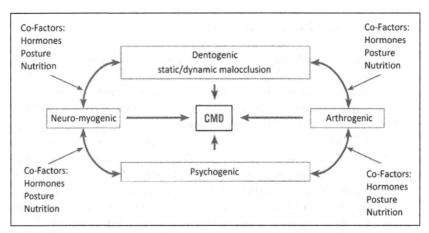

Figure 1.1:   Causes and co-factors which can lead to CMD in fluent transitions –
adapted from [57 P 125]. With kind permission by Quintessenz Verlags-
GmbH.

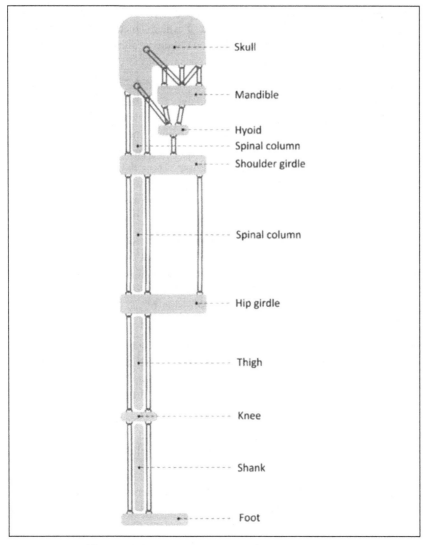

Figure 1.2: This extended Brody-Scheme shows the skeletal and muscular cybernetic interrelationships in CMS and MMS – adapted from [57 P 116]. With kind permission by Quintessenz Verlags-GmbH.

In general, increased muscle activity leads to an increase in metabolism with increased blood circulation through tissue, but also through bruxism. The mechanical properties of the connective tissue are modified to reduce the strain on the tendon, the collagen synthesis in the tendons themselves increasing. Adaptation always takes time. The resistance of the tissue to overload is increased [23]. If the load on the tissue is too great due to the elevated function-induced muscular activity, compensation is required. This condition is often not noticed by the patient, but in the functional diagnosis it is conspicuous as CMD [77].

If the compensation capacity is exhausted because the dysfunction or other disturbance factors persist or are not treated over time, the compensated function disorder develops a de-compensated function disorder, which is perceived by the patient as a disease with symptoms. If the decompensation progresses and is not treated, peripheral structures will also be detected by the dysfunction, which are often far from the primary triggering lesion. The relationships between the primary lesion and the acute pain elsewhere are increasingly difficult to detect, and interdisciplinary cooperation between dentistry and manual medicine is therefore indispensable [57].

Figure 1.3 shows an illustration of the so called "referred pain" as a special phenomenon relating to trigger points (TrPs). Trigger points arise from permanently strained muscle tissue after prolonged spasm or tension due to muscular hyperactivity. They may also be the result of a chronic or an acute traumatization. Active trigger points can lead to the transmission of pain into distant areas, to motor dysfunction, or to their own pain appearance [57].

The mutual influence of the craniomandibular and cranio-cervical system has been a subject of many other studies. Rocabado showed the influence of dysfunction of the cranio-cervical system with an altered posture of the head and neck on the retching of the lower jaw and thus also on the occlusion [78].

The effects of the occlusion on the hip-lumbar pelvic region in the sense of a craniosacral relationship have also been demonstrated [69,79]. In both studies occlusal changes by a few millimeters had an effect on the hip abduction or the function of the sacroiliac joint.

The study of Deregibus et al. handling electromyographically detectable hyperactivities in the trapezius and sternocleidomastoid muscles by malocclusion also supports the idea that the cranio-cervical system, the mandible of the lower jaw, the occlusion, and the craniosacral system are components of a large functional group, in which the change of a parameter always triggers adaptation mechanisms in the other functional areas [80]. This concept corresponds to the usual functional thinking of manual and osteopathic medicine [10].

A brief look at the nervous system could explain the previous chains as following: The convergence of proprioception in dental contact via the maxillary nerve and mandibular nerve with afferents from the dura mater on the spinal trigeminal nerves allows pain projection in the neck and head. The continuation of the spinal trigeminal nerve into the substantia gelatinosa of the spinal cord forwards the TMJ information to the spine. In addition, painful stimulation of trigeminal afferents leads to the triggering of postural reflexions on a segmental as well as supra-segmental level, which triggers a specific retention pattern [81]. Furthermore, cervical muscle afferents, in particular from C2 and C3, project into the complex of the vestibular nuclei and thus behave quite similar to the distribution patterns of the afferent tracts of the cerebral nerves Nn. Trigeminus, facialis, vagus and hypoglossus [82]. Stimuli that act on motoneurones or motor interneurons during short periods lead to persistent changes in motor basic functions which manifest themselves as a change in muscle tension, changes in posture, in particular asymmetry and limited mobility or pain [83].

According to Beyer, the location of the symptoms doesn't have to be identical with the origin of the triggering stimuli. If a portion is disturbed in a segment (sclerotome, myotome, dermatome, visceralotome), the disorder spreads over a sufficiently long period in the segment, then segmentally to the cranial and caudal, muscular, fascial and articulated chains of stereotypes. This spread does not take much time; often a couple of days. Manual therapists see, almost exclusively, such functionally linked symptoms (concatenation syndromes). In these cases, a "primary lesion" can usually no longer be identified. Thus, a treatment of the cerebral nerves area or the branches of the upper cervical nerves could reduce the muscle tension of the extremities and prevent asymmetries [82].

The functional interdependency between the craniomandibular, cranio-cervical, and craniosacral system, therefore, explains not only the origin of craniomandibular dysfunctions by the specific behavior of the violin, but leads also to a circular vitiosus due to the resulting tonus changes of the musculature overuse-syndromes [10].

The reason why professional violin playing is regarded as a possible predispositional factor for the development of a CMD lies in the specific behaviour of the violin. The instrument is braced between the left shoulder and the inferior border of the mandible, with the teeth often clenched to stabilize the mandible and prevent its deflection to the right. Although this pressure is captured by muscle contraction and teeth, but it can load and stress the temporomandibular joint and lead to its damage [31]. Prolonged application of pressure on the left mandible has also been considered a major cause of bruxism in violinists [51,84].

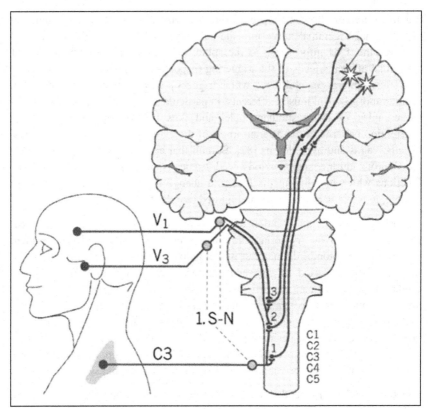

Figure 1.3: Pain in the temporomandibular joint can be caused by trapezius muscle, whereas frontal and parietal headache can have its cause in the temporomandibular joint. The information about C3 reaches from the active trigger point in the trapezius muscle to the second sensoneuron (2. SN) in the lower trigeminal nucleus under switching over in the first sensoneuron (1. SN). The first sensoneurons (1. SN) transport the information from the peripheral to the CNS. The information from the second sensoneuron (1) is transported to another sensoneuron (2) in the lower trigeminal nucleus. This sensoneuron (2) receives information not only from the trapezius muscle, but also from the temporomandibular joint. Here, the CNS cannot distinguish where the information comes from, so that the pain can be perceived in the CNS as TMJ pain. Due to the information divergence, the sensoneuron 3 receives two information; one from the temporomandibular joint via V3, the other from the dura mater via V1. Because of the higher receptor-density in the dura mater, the CNS cannot make a proper distinction, so that the pain is indicated as a headache, whereas the cause can be found in a TMJ-pathology. This is called a projection pain [57 P 105]. With kind permission by Quintessenz Verlags-GmbH.

Typical risk factors for the development of music-specific overloading problems (overuse syndromes) in violinists are as following [10]:

1) Sudden increase in playing time.

2) Psychological factors such as stress and stage fright.

3) Inadequate physical conditions, e.g. an inadequately trained musculature.

4) Poor biomechanical requirements.

5) Mistakes in training habits or instrument-specific techniques.

6) Workplace-related ergonomic aspects.

These result in increasing muscle tension during instrumental play, which subsequently leads to an overloading of the musculoskeletal system with the formation of an overload syndrome [85].

Other predisposing factors causing injuries in violinists include inefficient muscle use, poor posture, and poor techniques [86-88].

1.3.1 Biomechanical Aspects of the Violin

Quantitative biomechanical research into bowed string musicians has been performed with increasing frequency since 1983 [89]. During playing the violin, a pressure of between 30-70 Newton (5-14 N / cm²) and 220 and 2200 g is applied to the chin rest. The instrument makes a compressive pressure from the left lateral to the cranial and right lateral [4,90]. This causes compression of the right and subluxation of the left temporomandibular joint as an arthrogenic CMD cause, leading to degenerative changes in the right condylar head when the violin is held under the left side of the mandible for long periods of time. Furthermore, small repeated injuries can in some cases cause pathological remodeling of the right TMJ [10,43,91].

According to Hirsch et al., signs and symptoms resembling those of TMJ pain dysfunction syndrome that were found in violinists & violists are related to chronic irritations and mechanical displacement of the mandible by the position of the viola or violin, rather than to any active contraction of the jaw-closing muscles [44].

The two structures of a violin most likely to interface physically with the performer are the chin rest and the shoulder pad. They are among the factors cited in literature as possibly critical to the biomechanics of performance. Today, the chin rest is a standard part of the violin; with the exception of period Baroque players, the majority of violinists use some type of chin rest. There is no recorded evidence that today's commercially made chin rest were originally designed with systemic ergonomic principles in mind [4].

The use of an asymmetric type of chin rest (such as the Dresden model, in which the clamps and cup are on the left side of the instrument (Figure 1.4) has been demonstrated to be connected with deviation on opening of the mandible towards the side opposite that to which the violin is held when playing [91]. Signs and symptoms of TMJ disorders were revealed much less in violinists who used a "centered chinrest" than in those with a conventional side-positioned chinrest [44], whereas more painful mandibular movements were found in violinists who did not use any kind of shoulder support or a cushion-like-support [48].

Increasingly, music medicine specialists and performers are advising custom-made chin rests to optimize the ergonomic "fit" between the performer and the instrument [4]. Custom-made chin rests appear to reduce necessary holding pressure by spreading the load over a larger area, hence may have larger surfaces than the commercially available rests in addition to being custom-molded to the individual's jaw [92]. A custom-designed chin rest can improve head posture and distribute the force equally over the entire contact area, avoiding TMJ disorders [93].

Although chin rests were an early adaptation made to the violin, shoulder pads are a more common "ergonomic" device used in violin playing. Affixes to the back side of the instrument at its lower edge, the shoulder pads purpose is to aid the performer by achieving a more secure and thus more comfortable violin hold. Unlike chin rests, commercially made shoulder pads vary a great deal in size, shape, and material. Shoulder pads afford a better fit between musicians and their violins in several ways. The pad can fill the extra space between the chin and the shoulder. No matter what the size of the pad, it can provide the optimal friction between the instrument and the performers shoulder, so that the excessive slipping is prevented [4].

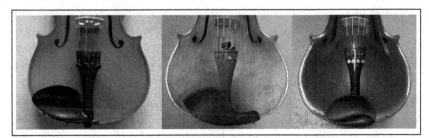

Figure 1.4:   The 3 types of chin rests. Dresden model (left), centered chinrest (right) – own photo.

1.3.2   Muscular Activity while Playing the Violin

Violin playing requires good function of the flexor muscles to stabilize the instrument [94]. In terms of the muscles involved in violin playing, the left upper trapezius (shoulder elevation) and right sternocleidomastoid muscle (SCM) (left cervical rotation and chin depression) together have a major role in holding the violin between the left shoulder and the chin [8]. While playing violin there is a shortening of the trapezius and the pectoralis major muscles against inhibited, weakened lower shoulder blade fixators and deep neck bugs. This leads to a head restraint position, which changes the resting position of the mandible [78].

Working with elevated arms leads to a high intramuscular pressure which impedes local muscle blood flow in the infraspinatus and supraspinatus muscles. A high intramuscular pressure causes reduced local blood flow in the muscles, which also affects the circulation in the muscle tendons, since blood perfusion in the tendon originates partly from the muscle. A reduced blood flow in combination with mechanical stress and a pinched muscular tendon could lead to degeneration, which causes pain, aching, and discomfort [28,95-98]. Furthermore, work tasks including repetitive work with the hands and arms demand an added amount of static load of the stabilizing scapular muscles, which could also lead to neck/ shoulder musculoskeletal disorders if executed during the majority of working time [99].

The scapula retractors, particularly the rhomboids and middle trapezius muscles, have an important role in providing scapula stability and thus in supporting the arm holding the instrument [100]. Scapulae and shoulders of violinists may become repositioned to be excessively protracted and elevated, especially on the left side. This forward and raised posture is associated with comparatively increased activity levels in the upper trapezius in relation to its middle and lower portions, and has been suggested to contribute to neck and upper limb injuries in these musicians [101,102]. In some violin players, the necessary static loading in the left shoulder required by long hours of violin playing and the repetitive loading of the left hand and right upper limb can cause muscular imbalances around the scapulae and shoulders, pain bilaterally in the upper limbs, and prolonged uneven loading of the cervical spine (in a left laterally rotated and flexed position), which may cause premature spinal degenerative changes [53].

Playing-related neck pain in violinists is also associated with changes in neuro-muscular control of cervical muscles and with altered behaviour of the superficial neck flexor muscles consistent with neck pain, despite the specific use of the deep and superficial neck flexors while playing [103].

The presence of such dysbalances can lead to development of CMD as a myogenic factor [10]. Perversely, CMD leads to an increase in muscle tension in the masticatory muscles as well as in peripheral muscles, like the shoulder-neck muscles [76]. Since an increase in the muscle tension during the play of violin can lead to overloading problems [85], it can be assumed that CMD can trigger overuse symptoms via this mechanism [10].

In a study aimed to confirm the presence of myofascial pain syndrome (MPS) in violinists, a high correlation was found between musculoskeletal pain and the presence of myofascial trigger points (MTrPs), and between hours of practice and number and severity of MTrPs. The muscles more frequently involved belonged to the cervical and scapular area and to the upper limb, with active MTrPs in upper trapezius, levator scapulae, left scalenus medius, left masseter, right latissimus dorsi, left triceps brachii, and latent MTrPs in sternocleidomastoid, right masseter, pectoralis minor, subscapularis, extensor carpi ulnaris, extensor carpi radialis longus and left dorsal interossei [104].

Furthermore, high amounts of practicing and playing hours are considered to be a risk factor for musculoskeletal disorders [35]. The number of hours of violin practice per week was positively correlated with selected signs of TMD. It was therefore concluded that violin playing could be a factor predisposing musicians to TMD [45].

1.3.3   Radiological Findings

There are only few papers discussing the influence of violin playing on bony facial structures in violinists. According to one study of Kovero et al. (1997) aiming to observe the effect of professional violin and viola playing on the bony facial structures, it was found that long-term professional violin playing has a modifying effect on dentofacial morphology. This effect was manifested as smaller facial heights, greater proclination of the maxillary incisors and greater length of the mandibular corpus in violin players than in controls. However, it seems that with regard to facial symmetry, the forces and pressures involved in violin playing are not unfavorable as they seem to reduce rather than increase facial asymmetry. Thus it could be assumed, that violin playing reduces growth of the facial height, but does not totally prevent it. Surprisingly, no statistically significant asymmetry of the face or the mandible was found in that study, although the instrument is pressed against the mandibular angle at the left, and the right condyle is pressed into the articular fossa during playing [49].

In a second study made by the same previous team in the same year, aiming to observe the effect of violin playing on the bony facial structures of adolescent violin players, it was revealed that the players had greater facial height measured from the PA Cephalogram and mild facial asymmetry with right-side dominance. The asymmetry was limited to the lower face. Both upper and lower incisors were more proclined in the players than in the controls. The reduced anterior and posterior facial heights seen in adult professional violin and viola players of the previous study [49] were not observed in the group of adolescent violin players of the second study, although the adolescents and professionals were similar with regard to the increased proclination of maxillary incisors. In the adolescent violinists there was a trend towards a more anteriorly rotated mandible, which may be an initial sign of the development leading to reduced anterior facial height. The finding in the violinist group of overall higher face and right-side dominance of the lower part of the face could be considered to result from playing the violin for many hours weekly, with the increased face muscle activity involve [105].

Kiliaridis (1995) found out that increased loading of the jaws due to masticatory muscle hyperfunction may lead to increased sutural growth and bone apposition, resulting in turn in an increased transversal growth of the maxilla and broader bone bases for the dental arches. Furthermore, an increase in the function of the masticatory muscles is associated with anterior growth rotation pattern of the mandible and with well-developed angular, coronoid, and condylar processes [106]. Holding the instrument under the left side of the chin induces balancing muscular activity on the right, and the playing position loads the right temporo-mandibular area. Thus, the etiology of the slight dominance of the right side of the lower face of the adolescent violinists may include increased functional activity [105]. This conclusion is also supported by the finding that the adolescent violinists had tenderness to palpation in their right lateral pterygoid muscle statistically significantly more often than controls in an investigation of signs and symptoms of temporomandibular disorders in adolescent violinists [48]. The increased proclination of the incisors could similarly be explained by an altered balance of muscular activity between the tongue and the lip, contributed by the pressure of the violin under the chin [105].

1.4 Diagnosis, Therapy and Prevention

There appears to be evidence for the contention that craniomandibular imbalances are prerequisite for playing a musical instrument professionally. For playing an instrument, all senses and muscles are needed. Total body balance achieved by the combination of posture, breathing, stability, and flexibility is essential. This can be easily disturbed by therapeutic intervention to correct CMDs disrupting the instrumental technique. So clinically, a distinction should be made between imbalances and dysfunctions. From a medical point of view, imbalances can in fact lead to problems, but musicians often do not suffer from that. Imbalances are to a certain extent an indispensable and necessary consequence of many years of practice to master the instrument till perfection [70].

Clinicians appreciate the full chain of tissue damage of the interconnecting muscles, tendons, ligaments and fascia: this compromised linkage from (1) The skull through the sub-occipital musculature to the cervical spine and anterior/ posterior cervical muscles, (2) from the check-rein ligaments and muscles extending from the skull and maxilla to the mandible, (3) from the suprahyoid musculature connecting the mandible through to the hyoid bone, (4) from the hyoid through the infrahyoid to the supporting shoulder girdle, all contribute to damaged interconnecting matrices. Consequently, unresolved tissue damage in any of this linkage becomes mutually provocative during function to any part of the linkage. Diagnostics, therefore, must necessarily include examination of this total linkage; similarly, eventual treatment protocols must resolve tissue damage in all of this interconnecting linkage if treatment is to be successful beyond palliative applications. Finally, if we are to treat the occlusion of these victims intelligently, we must understand the effects of a trauma on the 'whole body', and not just focus singularly on the restoration or the malocclusion or the TMJ problem. There are lessons to be learned from this acute trauma which provide valuable insights into the diagnosis of chronic pain patients. If these victims do not come for help immediately following the acute trauma episode, but arrive months or years later, the clinical examinations must include head and neck mobility or functional restrictions, observations of the patients' gait, and other residual postural deficits. Failure to implement these observations in our clinical examination will ultimately compromise our treatment success [107].

At medical offices, violinists should be questioned about the frequency and duration of their musical sessions. It is beneficial for them to demonstrate how their musical instruments are played. By observing and understanding how the instrument impacts on the orofacial structures, the therapist can gain a greater understanding of the patient's radiographs and study models [47]. Orthodontic consultation should also be proposed before starting to play an instrument and professional musicians should be offered prophylactic relaxation plates to avoid occurring dysfunction [55].

In a recent study, infrared thermal imaging (IRT) was used to evaluate the cutaneous thermal changes adjacent to the cranio-cervico-mandibular complex that occur before, during, and after playing a violin. It was suggested that these images could serve as a complementary examination to the clinical evaluation of musicians, because it could detect signs before they become complaints [108]. Infrared thermal imaging (IRT) is a non-invasive, non-contact technique which allows one to measure and visualize infrared radiation. In medicine, thermal imaging has been used for more than 50 years in various clinical settings, including Raynaud's phenomenon and systemic sclerosis. Despite certain limitations, thermal imaging can find a place in clinical practice, and with the introduction of small, low-cost infrared cameras, possibly become a part of routine rheumatic evaluation [109] (Figure 1.5).

The chain between the craniomandibular system (CMS) and the musculoskeletal system (MMS) is nowadays adequately described in the literature [10, 29, 63, 66, 110-117]. Thus, the CMS occupies a special position in the MMS, and functional disorders from the CMS have a dominant effect on the movement system in the sense of a primary lesion [118]. In return, patients with diseases of the musculoskeletal system have often concatenated problems with the CMS [119].

Generally, the therapy of CMD depends on its cause. In myogenic and occlusiongenic CMD, the therapy is usually a combination of occlusal splints with manual medicine, osteopathy and physiotherapy [10]. More and more patients undergoing dental treatment require interdisciplinary treatment concept. The dentist, orthodontist and implant surgeon should therefore collaborate with the chiropractor and the physiotherapist when treating patients with CMD. The endodontist and periodontist often need to be involved as well [119]. In the case of arthrogenic CMD, it is also possible in rare cases to undergo surgery by the surgeon, but methods of manual medicine or acupuncture are more successful because of their additional influence on the CMD-associated functional circles [10]. In complex chronic pain syndromes, accompanying psychotherapy is often necessary [120].

Violin playing can be a factor that predisposes or triggers the appearance of signs and symptoms of bruxism [51]. Clinical data from several researchers suggest that this bruxism could occur as a consequence of resisting an excessive shear force-related lateral shift of the mandible or habitual biting action with emotions [51,84,90]. So, reduction of lateral force can be of help in preventing TMJ problems, and an occlusal splint could be effective for protecting the teeth while clenching [51,84,121].

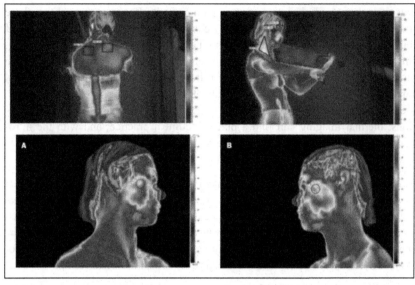

Figure 1.5:   Infrared thermal image (IRT) of a 32-year-old female violinist with one complaint: Soreness on the left side of her face involving the masseter region, showing temperature values in multiple zones such as TMJ, sterno-cleidomastoid, anterior temporalis, and masseter muscles of both right and left sides. Pictures A and B show differences in temperature values of left and right masseter regions of 0,9°C (more values in the left), making it possible to identify an asymmetric pattern of the left side compared to the right side of her face [108 P 253]. [1] With kind permission by Dr. Clemente M. et al., MPPA Journal and Science & Medicine, Inc.

Concerning occlusal splints, an evidence was provided on nonmusical subjects, revealing that an insertion of a 0.2-mm-thick occlusal interference positioned on a molar or premolar, provoked clear asymmetric activity in the masticatory and adjacent cervical muscles. Therefore, a small occlusal modulation could lead to a clear disturbance of normal functioning of the craniomandibular/ cervical system [122,123]. In violinists, it was observed that the inclusion of an adjusted bite can have a very positive effect [124]. Even the tinnitus associated with a CMD in some musicians was diminished after wearing occlusal splints [125,126].

Occlusal splints have a significant influence on the muscle tension not only of the masticatory muscles, but also of the shoulder-neck region and lower areas, even with highly complex motor performance, such as playing the violin [80]. This influence is also seen in asymptomatic violinists, suggesting a possible preventive

---

1   The coloured figure is also provided for free download on extras.springer.com.

and therapeutic role in the development of overuse symptoms in the setting of preexisting CMD. In particular, the effect of the splint on the sternocleidomastoid muscle and the trapezius muscle is to be estimated as very high for the prevention of overloading problems, since overuse complaints occur preferably in the shoulder region. Presumably, the altered resting iris and the suppression of the dysfunctional senso-motor input by using the splint lead to a neuromuscular reprogramming from the dysfunction [10].

A prerequisite for the successful manufacture of an occlusal splint is the adjustment of a new resting position of the mandible, in which the pathologies associated with the CMD, such as pelvic obliquity, disappear [10]. Reaching a new physiological resting position could take months and needs therefore multiple adjustment sessions at the dental office. The accompanying changes in the muscles and spine reached after physiotherapy will affect the cranium and thus also the lower jaw. So the occlusal splint has to be adjusted at regular intervals to the changed body situation [66,72]. These fine adjustments will also have an impact on the mobility of the cervical and lumbar spine [127]. At a later stage, a definite dental or orthodontic treatment of the occlusion can be connected [10].

Another treatment field for TMJ disorders and neck pain in violinists include the modification of the shoulder rest, physiotherapy and stress management [43].

Violinists and violists should also use a technique that reduces the force applied on the mandible by their instruments [44]. The Chin force develops laterally because of tilting of the neck and/or the violin. Therefore, raising the chinrest or the shoulder rest to the point in which the shoulder and neck approach neutral can help in the reduction of such force (Figure 1.6). It was also found that displacement of the chin rest to the center of the instrument "centered chinrest" can help to derotate the head and neck and will therefore have a very positive effect [124,128].

Even if the violinist isn't generating excessive pressure to hold the instrument, degenerative changes in the cervical spine can result from the abnormal posture of the head [53,129,130]. Brandfonbrener recommended the use of a shoulder pad to optimize the head and neck position as well as to alleviate tension in the shoulder. Muscle activity in the neck and shoulder area was measured during playing, with and without a shoulder pad. Electromyographic recordings showed that muscle activity changed as a result of the use of the shoulder pad. The results were predictable from neck and shoulder measurements, leading investigators to conclude that certain violinist may avoid musculoskeletal problems by utilizing a shoulder pad [8].

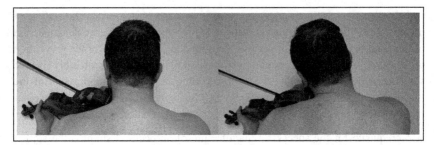

Figure 1.6:   Head position with a shoulder pad (left) and without it (right) – own photo.

Other researchers were also trying to observe the effects of using variations of shoulder rest height on the violinists' posture and movement. Complex and distributed body adaptations were observed, apparently managed by the anatomical parts involved in holding the violin (the left upper limb and head-trunk system); in particular, the left acromion elevation and a head leftward rotation compensates for a decreasing rest height. No significant adaptation was observed in the right upper limb holding the bow. In general, a variation of the rest height inversely affects the left upper limbs in relation to the other anatomical sectors, the former ones worsening while the latter improve and vice versa. These elements may help in the process of individually tuning the shoulder rest setup [131].

Other treatment options which also have been suggested as measures which have given some relief to violin players include altering posture, using a custom-made chin rest or padding of the chin rest, shorter practice times, placing a cloth between the instrument and the neck, resting the instrument on the clavicle, chewing sugar free gum during practice, and sitting rather than standing [43,129,132].

Playing positions have been discussed with regard to possible physiological stress and health risks. One study discussed unbalanced weight distributions while sitting in front of or oriented to the right of the music stand, and the analyses of the movement patterns showed significant differences between standing and sitting, mainly in the upper body parts with less movability while sitting. These findings emphasize the importance of different playing positions and offers starting points for discussion of postural influences and sensible handling of the instrument in performance and practice for violinists [133].

Many researchers have found that teaching better posture has a positive impact on TMJ health. Wright et al. performed a study to evaluate the efficiency of this approach. Seventy patients with TMD were chosen to take part and were randomly divided into 2 groups: One group received posture training and instruction in medical self-help for TMD, and the control group received only instruction in TMD self-help. Four weeks later, the authors examined the participants again and evaluated any changes that had taken place. They found an improvement in symptoms, painless mouth opening, and lower pain thresholds from pressure among the group that had received posture training. Thus, the playing position of the violin appears to be an important factor that should be considered in helping to minimize TMD [134].

The voluntary monitoring of shoulder muscle activity may be of great importance in the prevention of playing-related musculoskeletal disorders in violin players. A redistribution of the load to other synergistic muscles may be a strategy used to alleviate pain or discomfort at the neck-shoulder area [135]. This could be accomplished by Electromyography (EMG), which is one of the most commonly used tools allowing researchers to determine the amplitude and timing of muscle activation during instrumental performance, thus providing insight into playing-related injury mechanisms [89]. Using needle EMG, rather than surface EMG, on all major neck and shoulder muscles would enable a more specific measurement of muscle activity. Moreover, the possibility of controlling shoulder muscles voluntarily, and the trapezius muscle in particular, may be of great importance, and provide scope for development of EMG biofeedback as one of the prophylactic measures to consider in order to alleviate neck-shoulder muscle pain among violin players [135]. Currently, biofeedback can utilize EMG and displays muscular activity (often graphically or aurally). So the advantage is that it is an objective measure of muscle contraction that the player can use to correct improper techniques [89].

Since the anatomical and functional areas of the craniomandibular system are closely linked to the upper cervical spine, and the chain between the craniomandibular system (CMS) and the musculoskeletal system (MMS) is adequately described in the literature, the interdisciplinary collaboration between dentist, orthodontist and manual physician is an indispensable factor in the treatment of patients with CMD in general [30,136,137] and CMD-violinists in particular.

Furthermore, it is important to identify the other factors predisposing to disorders in violinists, such as sudden inadequate exercise routine, increase of playing sessions and rehearsal periods, as well as lack of warming-up and muscle stretching. Changing the posture or the instrument or the repertoire have also been mentioned. Other significant factors include individual and gender-related anatomical variability, improper chairs, extra-musical activities that produce muscle tension, quality of the instrument and the conditions of the room, with low lighting and temperature [2,138,139,140].

According to Ostwald et al., reduction of practice time, warming up prior to playing, incorporation of rest periods into training sessions, correcting problems of performing techniques, reduction of static and dynamic loads, physical or occupational therapy, ultrasonography, soft-tissue and neural mobilization, sensory and motor re-education, relaxation training, counseling psychotherapy, balanced diet and adequate hydration aid in managing musculoskeletal injuries in musicians [140].

According to Plato G. it is assured that CMD can only be safely and successfully treated in its initial stage. If the functional disturbances remain undetected and untreated for some time in the compensation phase, decompensated forms develop, not only the CMS, but gradually functional impairments in the entire musculoskeletal system. A chronic disease develops from a local dysfunction [77].

For the dental approach, peripheral manual tests allow conclusions to be made as to whether a descendant disorder originating from the CMS is present or whether this originates from the periphery (ascendant). If this is an exclusively ascendant problem the patient has to be treated by a manual medical technician. Only patients with a descendant or mixed problematic will be treated by dental and/or dentofacial orthopedic methods. A successful therapy is therefore only possible in an interdisciplinary cooperation. Using the manual tests and the change in the proprioception of the temporomandibular joints, both the dentist and the manual medical technician will be able to identify with certainty whether a chain is present and if the occlusion participates in the musculoskeletal disorder [119].

Therefore, any treatment strategy of CMD, especially in violinists, should be decided in an interdisciplinary collaboration between dental and manual medicine with paying a special attention to the violin playing as a predisposing factor for CMD.

2 Motivation and Aims

Craniomandibular Dysfunction (CMD) has a multifactorial etiology, such as physical trauma, parafunctional habits, anxiety and stress. All these have been suggested as important initiating and perpetuating factors.

Playing a musical instrument that loads the masticatory and cervical system like the violin, has been suggested to be part of the etiological factors of CMD. Therefore an up-to-date review of the literature to assess CMD among this highly risk group will indicate the extent of this problem, give an overview of diagnostic and therapeutic methods, sensitize practitioner dentists to a more accurate understanding of the unique work conditions of violinists and of all etiologic factors caused by playing this instrument, thus making dentists able to offer preventive advice and supportive treatment to violinists, especially for those in early stages of their career.

Moreover, the analysis of the included papers aims to reveal what exactly was studied in violinists regarding to CMD, and how far manual medicine was included there.

© Springer Fachmedien Wiesbaden GmbH, part of Springer Nature 2019
R. Abdunnur, *Craniomandibular Dysfunction in Violinists*,
https://doi.org/10.1007/978-3-658-24148-3_2

3   Material and Methods

A literature search of The National Library of Medicine's PubMed database was first performed on December 01.2016 and conducted without time restrictions, to retrieve all available articles in the literature written in both English and German language. Key words used in this search were (craniomandibular disorder) AND (violin). This search yielded twelve articles, eight of which were included in this review. Similar articles where gathered and reference lists of all articles were screened for other papers that might also be relevant and fulfil the inclusion criteria for this review and were retrieved in full texts. Furthermore, citation tracking was performed and more information were gathered from books published in German language dealing with musician specific diseases.

Papers that are included in the analysis are articles handling any form of diagnostic investigations and/or treatments performed on the upper and lower jaws, Temporomandibular Joints (TMJ), masticatory, shoulder, and cervical spine muscles of violin players suffering from CMD. Articles that did not fit the inclusion criteria were those performed on violists only, or on whole orchestras with poor results for violinists. Studies handling pure biomechanical aspects of the instrument without referring to CMD in violinists were also excluded. Likewise reviews, scoping studies and papers with only preliminary report.

© Springer Fachmedien Wiesbaden GmbH, part of Springer Nature 2019
R. Abdunnur, *Craniomandibular Dysfunction in Violinists*,
https://doi.org/10.1007/978-3-658-24148-3_3

4 Results

In the previous introduction, I was able to write an up-to-date literature review handling CMD in violinists, revealing it´s prevalence, signs and symptoms, etiology, predisposing factors, diagnosis, therapy and Prevention.

Concerning the following analysis, ten papers were identified for inclusion in this review. The final number of included studies that met the inclusion criteria is ten. They are divided into two groups, according to the type of the study. The first group contains five case-control papers and two pre-test-post-test studies. The second group contains three case reports. In the first group, four papers reveal the prevalence of TMD and its signs and symptoms, one paper measurs muscular load levels via quantitative EMG, one study shows the influence of CMD on shoulder-neck musculature and overuse syndromes, and the last paper applys oral splints as a treatment method.

The fiest group will be analysed according to the "PICO process" (stands for **P**opulation, **I**ntervention, **C**ontrol and **O**utcome) and the second group will be only summarised.

© Springer Fachmedien Wiesbaden GmbH, part of Springer Nature 2019
R. Abdunnur, *Craniomandibular Dysfunction in Violinists*,
https://doi.org/10.1007/978-3-658-24148-3_4

1. Hirsch JA, McCall WD, Bishop B. Jaw dysfunction in viola and violin players. 1982 [44]

Aim(s): To document:

1) Occurrence of pain, TMJ sounds and palpable crepitus, irregularities of mandibular movements and their relationship with the use of certain types of chinrests and shoulder pads.
2) Presence of deviation on maximal opening and its relationship with factors such as practice time, instrument weight and size.
3) Silent periods of the masseteric and right anterior temporalis muscles.

Population: Fifty-one professional violists and fifteen professional violinists, who had not sought after treatment for jaw problems, except one violist, who had been treated with a bite splint.

Intervention: Questioning, sEMG, recording of functional jaw movements via a small light bulb and an oscilloscope camera.

Control: 115 dental students who didn't had played violin or viola and had no history of TMJ pain dysfunction syndrome.

Outcome:

1) Maximal mouth opening was less in the musician's group than in the control group. It was also less in the violinists than in the violists.
2) Mandibular deviation was considerably more in the musician's group, with an obvious tendency to the right side while opening.
3) Size of mandibular deviation was related to the number of hours per week spent playing the instrument.
4) The left mandibular angle was palpably smoother than that of the right side.
5) TMJ pain and sounds were more often in the musician's group (pain located significantly in the right TMJ area whereas joint sounds in the left).
6) Prolonged EMG silent periods in the jaw closing muscles.
7) The frequency of pain and the size of deviation were significantly greater in violists than in violinists.

2. Philipson L, Sörbye R, Larsson P, Kaladjev S. Muscular load levels in performing musicians as monitored by quantitative electromyography. 1990 [85]

Aim(s)

1) Investigate the load level in various muscles in two groups of musicians.
2) Compare muscle load levels for different postures during performance:

A: standing without playing (rest).

B: sitting relaxed.

C: sitting tense.

D: standing relaxed playing détaché.

E: standing relaxed playing martellé.

Population: Five professional violinists with pain in neck and shoulder region (group 1).

Intervention: Bilateral sEMG recordings of the biceps, triceps, deltoid, and trapezius muscles.

Control: Four professional violinists without pain in neck and shoulder (group 0).

Outcome:

1) The grand mean NAREMG levels during rest (ID: A) were approximately equal for the two groups.
2) Different postures or activities (IDs: B, C, D and E) didn't significantly influence the grand mean NAREMG levels within the groups.
3) There was a significant difference between the groups in the grand mean NAREMG levels for IDs: B, C, D and E.
4) Musicians of group 1 showed a significantly higher NAREMG level in the left and right trapezius muscles. Besides, their right deltoids and right biceps were significantly more involved.

3. Kovero O, Könönen M. Signs and symptoms of temporomandibular disorders and radiologically observed abnormalities in the condyles of the temporomandibular joints of violin and viola players. 1995 [45]

Aim(s): Investigate whether professional violin and viola players have more signs and symptoms of TMD or radiologically observed abnormalities in the condyles of the TMJs of and their controls.

Population: Sixteen violinists and ten violists, who were not diagnosed as having any general joint diseases (VP group: The violinist-violist Players).

Intervention:

1) Routine stomatognathic examination and personal interview
2) Examination of mandibular mobility with a ruler, recording of: TMJ noises, painful mandibular movements and occlusal relations.
3) Palpation of the TMJs, masticatory, sternocleidomastoid, trapezius, deltoid and greater pectoral muscles and recording the tenderness score for each muscle.
4) Panoramic examination of the TMJs using a TMJ program.

Control: Twenty six patients receiving regular dental treatments and don't play violin or viola (C group).

Outcome:

1) An association between muscle symptoms and intense playing was reported by 22 of 26 players.
2) The (VP) group had palpatory tenderness in their masticatory muscles more often than controls (C). Only the left-side differences was significant.
3) The difference in palpatory tenderness of the muscles was significant for the left deep masseter, left medial pterygoid, left lateral pterygoid and left deltoid muscles.
4) The (VP) group showed deviation on movement twice as often as the (C) group.
5) The deviation in the (VP) group was more often to the right.
6) Painful mandibular movements and audible clicks were found more often in the (VP) group.
7) No statistically significant difference in the radiologic findings between the groups (abnormality of shape, sclerosis of the joint and osteophyte formation)
8) Weekly playing hours correlated significantly with the TMJ pain during movement. Also, right-sided clicking and locking were significantly correlated.

4. Kovero O, Könönen M. Signs and symptoms of temporomandibular disorders in adolescent violin players. 1996 [48]

Aim(s): Investigate the frequency of radiologically observed abnormalities in the condyles of the TMJs of adolescent violin players (VP) and their controls (C).

Population: Thirty one adolescent violin players, eight of them were receiving or had received orthodontic treatment. None of them had grave facial asymmetries or malocclusions.

Intervention:

1) Routine stomatognathic examination.
2) Personal review concerning TMJ pain, playing and the individual instrument (type of chin rest and shoulder support).
3) Measurement of mandibular mobility with a ruler and recording of TMJ noises, painful mandibular movements and deviations (2 mm or more), occlusal relations, overbite & overjet.
4) Palpation of the TMJs, masticatory, sternocleidomastoid, trapezius, deltoid, greater pectoral and the upper limbs muscles.
5) Panoramic examination of the TMJs using a TMJ program.

Control: Thirty one children receiving general dental or orthodontic treatment. None of them had grave facial asymmetries or grave malocclusions and none had played a violin.

Outcome:

1) The number of subjective symptoms of TMD was greater in the (VP) group than in the (C) group. The symptoms were more severe and were statistically significant in: TMJ-Pain on chewing, stiffness in the TMJs and clenching of teeth.
2) The (VP) group showed: Greater range of maximal protrusion, greater range of maximal laterotrusion to the right, greater frequency of tenderness to palpation in the muscles palpated with statistically significant difference only for the right lateral pterygoid muscle and the left trapezius muscle, more pain in TMJs on maximal opening.
3) Radiologic findings in the condyles were statistically not significant.
4) Positive correlation between the type of the violins shoulder support and painful mandibular movements (more pain without a support or only a cushion-support).

5. Steinmetz A, Ridder P-H, Reichelt A. Influence of craniomandibular dysfunction on the shoulder neck muscles of violinists. 2005 [10]

Aim(s): Investigate the frequency of CMD among the examined violinists, analog to the studies of Hirsch, Kovero and Könönen, and whether CMD can cause overuse symptoms in violinists.

Population: Thirty one violinists.

Intervention:

Questionnaire, analysis of the jaw function via "zebris JMA", clinical examination (orthopedically and manually) to evaluate overuse and CMD symptoms, assess the influence of CMD on muscle tension during violin playing via four canal surface EMG "myosys o1 easy, Fa. mediTronic, Jena" (applied both with and without an individual occlusal splint). The evaluating software was "EMG Utils".

Control: No control group.

Outcome:

1) Overuse syndrome in 74 % of the violinists.
2) CMD in 70 %.
3) Pain while playing in 81 %.
4) Pain while clinical examination in 39 %.
5) Pain while palpating the masticatory muscles in 65 %.
6) Pain was most frequently located in the areas of the right shoulder, cervical and lumbar spine.
7) Pain in TMJ 16 %.
8) TMJ noises in 58 %.
9) Maximum mouth opening less than 41 mm in 87 %.
10) Deviation of the mandible in 93 % (63 % to the right and 30 to the left).
11) Functional dysbalances in 81 % in form of: Weakening of the neck flexors (58 %), forward flexion phenomenon (52 %), functional reduction of leg length (39 %), face scoliosis (39 %), cymbal twisting (16 %)
12) Michigan splints significantly reduced EMG values: Most significantly in the masseter, followed by temporalis, trapezius, sternocleidomastoid, and extensors muscles.

6.   Steinmetz A, Ridder P-H, Methfessel G, Muche B. Professional Musicians with Craniomandibular Dysfunctions Treated with Oral Splints. 2009 [75]

Aim(s): Investigate the effect of oral splint treatment of CMD on reducing pain and symptoms in the neck, shoulders and arms of violin/viola playres.

Population: Thirty professional musicians (including 11 violinists and 3 violists) who were all under interdisciplinary orthopedic and dental care. The majority were known to have had several unsuccessful attempts at treatment before being diagnosed with TMD. They had the following criteria:

1) Myofacial pain in the masticatory muscles (spontaneous or upon palpation).
2) Restricted mouth opening (<40 mm).
3) Deviation or deflection on opening.
4) Pain within the TMJ upon palpation or during mouth movements.
5) Malocclusion (Angles II and III).

Intervention:

1) Questionnaire asking about TMD symptoms, pain regions and severity, occurrence of symptoms while playing the instrument and its influence on the musician's ability to perform, and therapy results.
2) Michigan splint in the lower jaw being adjusted in the mouth in centric position with canine guidance to be used at night and while playing the instrument.
3) Software (SPSS/PC for windows Inc., Chicago, IL, USA) for statistical analysis.

Control: No control group.

Outcome:

1) Nocturnal bruxism diagnosed by dental practitioner was evidenced in 16 musicians (53 %); two (7 %) denied the presence of bruxism, whereas 12 (40 %) denied self-awareness of it.
2) 80 % of the musicians experienced a significant improvement in symptoms by wearing the splint.
3) 20 % reported a decrease in the number of days they weren't able to play their instrument.
4) Pain increased again in 40 % of the musicians when not wearing the splint.

7. Rodríguez-Lozano FJ, Sáez-Yuguero MR, Bermejo-Fenoll A. Prevalence of temporomandibular disorder-related findings in violinists compared with control subjects. 2010 [52]

Aim(s): Study the prevalence of signs and symptoms of TMD in a group of musicians and analyse differences between men and women in the results. Determine whether musicians were aware of the existence of these pathologies as related to playing the violin, and if there is an association between signs and symptoms of TMD and the number of hours or years of practice.

Population: Fourty-one professional and semi-professional violinists who didn't have antecedents of TMD or had received orthodontic treatment.

Intervention:

1) Questionnaire (RCD/TMD).
2) Clinical examination in form of muscle palpation (to locate trigger points and hypertrophy in masseter and temporalis), auscultation of the TMJ, assessing the presence and intensity of pain during jaw opening with a visual analog scale calibrated from 1 to 10, measurement of mouth opening, measurement of the extent and protrusion of lateral movements.
3) Radiograph (OPG) to evaluate any pathologic finding that could affect the clinical examination, especially of the TMJ.
4) Software package SPSS 15.0 for statistical analysis.

Control: Fifty healthy subjects who had not previously attended dental school or played a musical instrument. They had neither orthodontic complaints nor were aware of having signs and symptoms of TMD.

Outcome:

1) The violinists group had more pain on maximum mouth opening, more TMJ sounds, and more parafunctional habits.
2) Only two musicians knew about the existence of TMD and its potential relationship with playing the violin.
3) No abnormal radiological findings could be observed in both groups.
4) No relationship between signs and symptoms of TMD and weekly hours or number of years of practice.
5) No significant gender difference of TMD signs and symptoms, although five relevant indicators of TMD were more prevalent in the women than the men, and pain in maximum opening approached statistical significance.

8. Rieder CE. Possible premature degenerative temporomandibular joint disease in violinists. 1976 [50]

Patient: 20-year-old white female violinist. Occasional discomfort in the right TMJ region. Mandibular deflection to the right side on opening. Right TMJ clicking with movement. Pain in the right TMJ upon palpation. Habitual clenching of jaw muscles and chronic headaches. Some discomfort in both right and left lateral pterygoid and sternomastoid muscles. Severely reduced right TMJ space with condylar irregularities were seen on radiographs.

Diagnosis: Premature TMJ degeneration with no systemic factors.

9. Kovero O. Degenerative temporomandibular joint disease in a young violinist. 1989 [91]

Patient: 11-year-old boy who played the violin since the age of 6 for 10-13 h/ week. Angles Class II Division 1 malocclusion. Deviation of mandible to the right side with maximal opening. Occasional discomfort with mouth opening in the morning. Episodes of acute otitis media. The panoramic radiograph showed a broader and flatter right condylar head in comparison with the left side and apparent loss of the articular eminence. Marked difference in heights of mandibular angles was seen on the lateral cephalometric radiograph. A tender posterior part of the right temporal muscle to palpation. Slightly painful right TMJ.

Diagnosis: Advanced degeneration in the right TMJ with no evidence for trauma or systemic disease.

10. Ward MR. Myofascial pain in a young violin player. 1990 [141]

Patient: 17-year-old female violin player who had undergone orthodontic therapy leaving occlusal interferences which were initially able to be tolerated. Early clicks on both TMJs on opening and closing. Jaw locked close periodically. Noticeable protrusion of the mandible while playing the violin.

Treatment and outcome: Provision of segmental bite plane, which was worn at night as required. Patient was comfortable at succeeding visits, but with persistent clicks. After 15 months, Patient was under stress and presented with pain in the left TMJ region. Bite plane was replaced with Michigan splint to be worn continuously until the patient become symptom free. After 1 week, the clicks were absent and the patient comfortable.

5 Discussion and Conclusion

According to the previous results, clinical signs and symptoms were more frequent in violinists than in controls; more TMJ sounds and pain, smaller and more painful maximum mouth opening and more parafunctional habits (1, 3, 4, 7). Concerning the mandible deviation on opening, there were more deviations to the right side, whereas violinists who played left-handed (the instrument was held on the right side) had mandibular deviations toward the left side, reported pain in the left TMJ area and had joint noises with stiffness in the right TMJ area. This was the mirror image of the signs observed in the right-handed players (1). Radiographic abnormalities in the TMJs were not present (3, 4). Degenerative changes after long periods of violin playing were found in two case reports (8, 9).

Etiologically, it was concluded that signs and symptoms are similar to those of TMJ pain dysfunction syndrome and are related to chronic irritations and mechanical displacement of the mandible by the position of the violin, rather than to any active contraction of the jaw-closing muscles (1). A violinist's mandible tends to be pushed towards the contralateral TMJ, thus mechanical overloads on that TMJ and musculature are formed (4, 5, 6). There was no significant influence of different postures of the violinists on the load level of various muscles investigated (2). Concerning shoulder pads, it was found that not using a shoulder support or using a cushion-support will create more muscular activity in order to bring the chin and shoulder closer together when holding the instrument, resulting in a positive correlation between the type of shoulder supports and painful mandibular movements (4). Concerning chin reasts, signs and symptoms of TMJ disorders were revealed much less in violinists who used a "centered chin rest" than in those with a conventional side-positioned chin rest (1). A violin's dimension was an important factor affecting the playing position, thus TMDs (4). The size of mandibular deviation and the number of playing hours were positively correlated. Besides, playing hours were significantly correlated with TMJ pain, and an association between muscle symptoms and intense violin playing was also found (1, 3, 4).

Compliance to the treatment with oral splints was high with a positive influence in reducing muscular load and TMJ clicks, showing an important improvement of pain intensity and pain frequency. It has been suggested, that these splints have a possible preventive and therapeutic role in the development of overuse symptoms in case of pre-existing CMD (5, 6, 10).

© Springer Fachmedien Wiesbaden GmbH, part of Springer Nature 2019
R. Abdunnur, *Craniomandibular Dysfunction in Violinists*,
https://doi.org/10.1007/978-3-658-24148-3_5

It was recommended that violinists should use a technique that reduces the force on the mandible by the instrument (1) and should receive routine occlusal and TMJ examinations as well as adequate therapies, especially those with musculoskeletal problems (5, 6, 8). It was mentioned that providing them with health education programs to investigate whether education and preventive measures help them to reduce the prevalence of TMD manifestations would also be very beneficial (7).

In addition to the former analysed articles, I found three interesting literature reviews handling related topics with similar results:

The first one is a systematic review accomplished by de Souza Moraes and Antunes, aiming to identify the musculoskeletal disorders that most frequently affect professional violinists and violists. In their study it was concluded that neck, shoulder and temporomandibular joint are the most commonly affected areas due to prolonged flexion of the head and shoulder required to hold the violin. This position could affect the cervical spine causing muscle spasms and nerve compression. They suggested to warn musicians of the initial symptoms, and show them how they can prevent such disorders from worsening. Incorrect postures, improper methods and considerable discrepancy between the size of the musician and violin should be avoided and corrected. Maintenance of the instrument and appropriate use of furniture should also not be ignored [142].

The second one is a literature review by Atallah MM. et al., searching for a possible association between playing a musical instrument and developing and/or having a TMD. All their included articles suggested a possible association between TMD and playing a musical instrument, especially the violin and viola. They mentioned that no clear-cut conclusion could be drawn as to whether playing a musical instrument is directly associated with TMD, or only in combination with other factors. Thus they suggested more and better research on this topic, as to enable a better counselling and possibly even a better treatment of the suffering musician [143].

The third one is an evidence-based review by van Selms MKA et al, aiming to investigate whether playing a musical instrument or singing increases the risk of developing TMDs. Based on their available evidence, the purported relationship between playing specific musical instruments and TMDs was not as evident as reported in previous literature reviews. An inconclusive evidence to support the assertion that "musicians playing an instrument that loads the masticatory system and neck region report TMDs more frequently" was attained in their study. In their paper, studies that investigated the presence of TMDs among violists and violinists yielded ambiguous outcomes; some of them reported no association between playing these instruments and the presence of signs and symptoms of TMDs, whereas in studies where a clinical examination was performed, an association was found. The authors referred to "TMJ sounds" as the only common thing in these clinical studies and suggested well-designed cohort or large-scale cross-sectional studies to be performed in the future to achieve a better evaluation [144].

According to the main results of the ten articles I've analysed here, I can say that a general agreement that violin playing is a predisposing factor in the etiology of CMD exists. Based on the literature review that I've accomplished previously in my introduction, I could find other worthy studies discussing the biomechanical effects of playing the violin on specific body regions of asymptomatic violinists. Since a close linkage between the anatomical and functional areas of the craniomandibular system (CMS) and the musculoskeletal system (MMS) has been adequately described in the literature, it can be well understood, that the influence of intense violin playing, as a prolonged asymmetrical position of the body, could lead to pathologic changes in both systems with time. Studies handling this linkage in symptomatic violinists are yet rare. More researches which take the interdisciplinary collaboration between dental and manual medicine into special account are therefore recommended. Only then, a well-structured diagnostic modality and better therapy standards could be obtained for those highly risk patients.

References

(1)   Zaza C, Charles C, Muszynski A. The meaning of playing-related musculoskeletal disorders to classical musicians. Soc Sci Med. 1998; 47(12):2013-23.

(2)   Winold H, Thelen E, Ulrich BD. Coordination and Control in the Bow Arm Movements of Highly Skilled Cellists. Ecol Psychol. 1994; 6(1):1-31.

(3)   Ericsson KA, Charness N. Expert Performance: Its Structure and Acquisition. Am Psychol. 1994; 49(8):725-47.

(4)   Okner MAO, Kernozek T, Wade MG. Chin rest pressure in violin players: musical repertoire, chin rests and shoulder pads as possible mediators. Med Probl Perform Art. 1997; 12(4):112-21.

(5)   Guptill C, Golem MB. Case study: musicians' playing-related injuries. Work. 2008; 30(3):307-10.

(6)   Hoppmann RA, Reid RR. Musculoskeletal problems of performing artists. Curr Opin Rheumatol. 1995; 7(2):147-50.

(7)   Heinan M. A review of the unique injuries sustained by musicians. JAAPA. 2008; 21(4):45-50.

(8)   Levy CE, Lee WA, Brandfonbrener AG, Press J, Levy AE. Electromyographic analysis of muscular activity in the upper extremity generated by supporting a violin with and without a shoulder rest. Med Probl Perform Art. 1992; 7(4):103-9.

(9)   Menuhin Y. The Violin. 1st edition. Paris: Flammarion. 1996.

(10) Steinmetz A, Ridder P-H, Reichelt A. Kraniomandibuläre Dysfunktionen und deren Einfluss auf die Schulter-Nacken-Muskulatur bei Geigern. Manuelle Medizin. 2005; 43(4):249-56.

(11) Kaufman-Cohen Y, Ratzon R. Correlation between risk factors and musculoskeletal disorders among classical musicians. Occup Med. 2011; 61(2):90-5.

(12) Kok LM, Huisstede BMA, Voorn VMA, Schoones JW, Nelissen RGHH. The occurrence of musculoskeletal complaints among professional musicians: a systematic review. Int Arch Occup Environ Health. 2016; 89(3):373-96.

(13) American Academy of Orofacial Pain. In: de Leeuw R [ed]. Orofacial Pain: Guidelines for assessment, diagnosis and management. 4th edition. Chicago: Quintessence. 2008.

(14) Heikinheimo K, Salmi K, Myllärniemi S, Kirveskari P. A longitudinal study of occlusal interferences and signs of craniomandibular disorders at the ages of 12 and 15 years. Eur J Orthod. 1990; 12(2):190-7.

(15) Hirata RH, Heft MW, Hernandez B, King GJ. Longitudinal study of signs of temporomandibular disorders (TMD) in orthodontically treated and non-treated groups. Am J Orthod Dentofac Orthop. 1992; 101(1):35-40.

(16) Sadowsky C. The risk of orthodontic treatment for producing temporomandibular disorders: a literature overview. Am J Orthod Dentofac Orthop. 1992; 101(1):79-83.

(17) Agerberg G, Carlsson GE. Functional disorders of the masticatory system: Distribution of symptoms according to age and sex as judged from investigation by questionnaire. Acta Odontol Scand. 1972; 30(6):597-613.

© Springer Fachmedien Wiesbaden GmbH, part of Springer Nature 2019
R. Abdunnur, *Craniomandibular Dysfunction in Violinists*,
https://doi.org/10.1007/978-3-658-24148-3

(18) Magnusson T, Carlsson GE. Comparison between two groups of patients in respect of headache and mandibular dysfunction. Swed Dent J. 1978; 2(3):85-92.

(19) Graber G. Neurologische und psychosomatische Effekte der Myoarthropathie des Kauorgans. Zahnärztl Welt. 1971; 80:997.

(20) Heggendorn H, Vogt HP, Graber G. Experimentelle Untersuchungen über die orale Hyperaktivität bei psychischer Belastung, im Besonderen bei Aggression. Schweiz Monatsschr Zahnmed. 1979; 89(11):1148-61.

(21) Csernay A, Graber G, Pfändler U. Psycho-emotionaler Einfluss auf die Funktionen des stomatognathen Systems – eine Studie an Untersuchungsgefangenen. Schweiz Monatsschr Zahnmed. 1984; 94(4):274-89.

(22) Geissler PR. Welche Rolle spielt Stress? Mandibuläres Dysfunktionssyndrom. J Dent. 1985; 13:283.

(23) Graber G. Der Einfluss von Psyche und Stress bei funktionsbedingten Erkrankungen des stomatognathen Systems. 1. Auflage. München: Urban und Schwarzenberg. 1995.

(24) Fjellman-Wiklund A, Sundelin G. Musculoskeletal discomfort of music teachers: an eight-year perspective and psychosocial work factors. Int J Occup Environ Health. 1998; 4(2):89-98.

(25) Sataloff R, Brandfonbrener A, Lederman R. Textbook of Performing Arts Medicine. 2nd edition. San Diego: Singular Publishing Group. 1998.

(26) Fjellman-Wiklund A, Grip H, Karlsson JS, Sundelin G. EMG trapezius muscle activity pattern in string players: part I - is there variability in the playing technique? Int J Ind Ergon. 2004; 33(4):347-56.

(27) Fjellman-Wiklund A, Chesky K: Musculoskeletal and general health problems of acoustic guitar, electric guitar, electric bass and banjo players. Med Probl Perform Art. 2006; 21(4):169-76.

(28) Edling CW, Fjellman-Wiklund A. Musculoskeletal disorders and asymmetric playing postures of the upper extremities and back in music teachers - a pilot study. Med Probl Perform Art. 2009; 24(3):113-8.

(29) Hansson T, Honneé l, Hesse J. Einige biomechanische Relationen im Kopf-Hals-Gebiet. In: Hansson T [Hrsg]. Funktionsstörungen im Kausystem. 2. Auflage. Heidelberg: Hüthig Medizin. 1990.

(30) Schupp W. Kraniomandibuläre Dysfunktionen und deren periphere Folgen - eine Literaturübersicht. Manuelle Medizin. 2005; 43(1):29-33.

(31) Spahn C, Richter B, Altenmüller E. Musiker Medizin - Diagnostik, Therapie und Prävention von musikerspezifischen Erkrankungen. 1. Auflage. Stuttgart: Schattauer. 2011.

(32) Silva AG, Filipa MB, Lã VA. Pain prevalence in instrumental musicians: A systemic review. Med Probl Perform Art. 2015; 30(01):8-19.

(33) Steinmetz A, Scheffer I, Esmer E, Delank KS, Peroz I. Frequency, severity and predictors of playing-related musculoskeletal pain in professional orchestral musicians in Germany. Clin Rheumatol. 2015; 34(5):965-73.

(34) Nyman T, Wiktorin C, Mulder M, Johansson YL. Work postures and neck-shoulder pain among orchestra musicians. Am J Ind Med. 2007; 50(5):370-6.

(35) Hagberg M, Thiringer G, Brandström L. Incidence of tinnitus, impaired hearing and musculoskeletal disorders among students enrolled in academic music education - a retrospective cohort study. Int Arch Occup Environ Health. 2005; 78(7):575-83.

(36) Lockwood AH. Medical problems of musicians. N Engl J Med. 1989; 320(4):221-7.

(37) Zaza C, Farewell VT. Musicians' playing-related musculoskeletal disorders: an examination of risk factors. Am J Ind Med. 1997; 32(3):292-300.

(38) Fishbein M, Middlestadt SE, Ottati V, Straus S, Ellis A. Medical problems among ICSOM musicians: overview of a national survey. Med Probl Perform Art. 1988; 3(1):1-4.

(39) Middlestadt SE, Fishbein M. The prevalence of severe musculoskeletal problems among male and female symphony orchestra string players. Med Probl Perform Art. 1989; 4(1):41-8.

(40) Fry HJ. Incidence of overuse syndrome in the symphony orchestra. Med Probl Perform Art. 1986; 1(2):51-5.

(41) Hiner SL, Brandt KD, Katz BP, French RN, Beczkiewicz TJ. Performance-related medical problems among premier violinists. Med Probl Perform Art. 1987; 2:67-71.

(42) Taddey JJ. Musicians and temporomandibular disorders: prevalence and occupational etiologic considerations. Cranio. 1992; 10(3):241-4.

(43) Zimmers PL, Gobetti JP. Head and neck lesions commonly found in musicians. J Am Dent Assoc. 1994; 125(11):1487-96.

(44) Hirsch JA, McCall WD, Bishop B. Jaw dysfunction in viola and violin players. J Am Dent Assoc. 1982; 104(6):838-43.

(45) Kovero O, Könönen M. Signs and symptoms of temporomandibular disorders and radiologically observed abnormalities in the condyles of the temporomandibular joints of violin and viola players. Acta Odontol Scand. 1995; 53(2):81-4.

(46) Carlsson GE. Epidemiology and treatment need for temporomandibular disorders. J Orofac Pain. 1999; 13(4):232-7.

(47) Yeo D, Pham T, Baker J, Porter S. Specific Orofacial Problems Experienced by Musicians. Aust Dent J. 2002; 47(1):2-11.

(48) Kovero O, Könönen M. Signs and symptoms of temporomandibular disorders in adolescent violin players. Acta Odontol Scand. 1996; 54(4):271-4.

(49) Kovero O, Könönen M, Pirinen S. The effect of professional violin and viola playing on the bony facial structures. Eur J Orthod. 1997; 19(1):39-45.

(50) Rieder CE. Possible premature degenerative temporomandibular joint disease in violinists. J Prosthet Dent. 1976; 35(6):662-4.

(51) Rodríguez-Lozano FJ, Sáez-Yuguero MR, Bermejo-Fenoll A. Bruxism related to violin playing. Med Probl Perform. 2008; 23(1):12-5.

(52) Rodríguez-Lozano FJ, Sáez-Yuguero MR, Bermejo-Fenoll A. Prevalence of temporomandibular disorder-related findings in violinists compared with control subjects. Pathol Oral Radiol Endod. 2010; 109(1):e15-e9.

(53) Fry HJ. Overuse syndrome in musicians: Prevention and management. The Lancet 1986; 2(8509):728-31.

(54) Lederman RJ, Calabrese LH. Overuse syndrome in instrumentalists. Med Probl Perform Art. 1986; 1:7-11.

(55) Głowacka A, Matthews-Kozanecka M, Kawala M, Kawala B. The impact of the long-term playing of musical instruments on the stomatognathic system - review. Adv Clin Exp Med. 2014; 23(1):143-6.

(56) Selye H. The stress of life. 1st edition. New York: McGraw-Hill. 1956.

(57) Boisserée W, Schupp W. Kraniomandibuläres und Muskuloskelettales System: Funktionelle Konzepte in der Zahnmedizin, Kieferorthopädie und Manualmedizin. 1. Auflage. Berlin: Quintessenz Verlag. 2012.

(58) Derbolowski U. Schmerzsyndrome aus psychsomatischer Sicht. In: Dittel R [Hrsg]. Schmerzphysiotherapie. 1. Auflage. Stuttgart, Jena, New York: Gustav Fischer Verlag. 1992.

(59) Amorim MIT, Jorge AIL. Association between temporomandibular disorders and music performance anxiety in violinis. Occup Med. 2016; 66(7):558-63.

(60) Mohlin B, Thilander B. The importance of the relationship between malocclusion and mandibular dysfunction and some clinical applications in adults. Eur J Orthod. 1984; 6(3):192-204.

(61) Mohlin B, Ingervall B, Thilander B. Relation between malocclusion and mandibular dysfunction in Swedish men. Eur J Orthod. 1990; 2(4):229-38.

(62) Egermark I, Thilander B. Craniomandibular disorders with special reference to orthodontic treatment: an evaluation from childhood to adulthood. Am J Orthod Dentofac Orthop. 1992; 101(1):28-34.

(63) Steinmetz A, Ridder P-H, Reichelt A. Craniomandibuläre Dysfunktionen als ein Einflussfaktor für die Entstehung von Überlastungsbeschwerden bei Geigern. Musikphysiol und Musikermed. 2003; 10(4):203-9.

(64) Droschl H, Permann I, Bantleon HP. Changes in occlusion and condylar positioning during retention with a gnathologic positioner. Eur J Orthod. 1989; 11(3):221-7.

(65) Koike H, Yamashita S, Hashii K, Nakatsuka Y, Mizoue S, Tomida M, et al. Relationship between condylar displacement during clenching and condylar inclination. Nihon Hotetsu Shika Gakkai Zasshi. 2007; 51(3):546-55.

(66) Ridder P-H. Kieferfunktionsstörungen und Zahnfehlstellungen mit ihren Auswirkungen auf die Körperperipherie. Manuelle Medizin. 1998; 36(4):194-212.

(67) Seidel EJ, Methfessel G, Günther P. Craniomandibuläre Dysbalancen als Technikvoraussetzung bei Bläsern. Phys Med Rehab Kur. 2001; 11(4):151.

(68) Kopp S, Plato G, Sebald WG. Was Musiker und deren Ärzte vom "Kiefergelenk" des Menschen wissen sollten. In: Seidel E, Lange E [Hrsg]. Die Wirbelsäule des Musikers. Schriftenreihe des Institutes für Musikpädagogik und Musiktheorie der Hochschule für Musik Weimar. Bad Kösen: GFBB-Verlag. 2001. S. 56-74.

(69) Fink M, Tschernitschek H, Wähling K, Stiesch-Scholz M. Einfluss okklusaler Veränderungen auf die Funktion der Wirbelsäule. ZWR. 2004; 113(07/08):314-21.

(70) Günther P, Zima K, Seidel EJ. Kraniomandibuläre Dysbalancen als Voraussetzung für professionelle Leistungen am Musikinstrument? Manuelle Medizin. 2005; 43(4): 243-48.

(71) Köneke C. Die interdisziplinäre Therapie der Craniomandibulären Dysfunktion. 1. Auflage. Berlin: Quintessenz. 2005.

(72) Ahlers MO, Jakstat HA. Klinische Funktionsanalyse. Interdisziplinäres Vorgehen mit optimierten Befundbögen. 3. Auflage. Hamburg: dentaConcept. 2007.

(73) Stiesch-Scholz M, Fink M, Tschernitschek H. Comorbidity of internal derangement of the temporomandibular joint and silent dysfunction of the cervical spine. J Oral Rehabil. 2003; 30(4):386-91.

(74) Pallegama RW, Ranasinghe AW, Weerasinghe VS. Influence of masticatory muscle pain on electromyographic activities of cervical muscles in patients with myogenous temporomandibular disorders. J Oral Rehabil. 2004; 31(5):423-9.

(75) Steinmetz A, Ridder P-H, Methfessel G, Muche B. Professional Musicians with Craniomandibular Dysfunctions Treated with Oral Splints. Cranio. 2009; 27(4):221-30.

(76) Ehrlich R, Garlick D, Ninio M. The effect of jaw clenching on electromyographic activities of 2 neck and 2 trunk muscles. J Orofac Pain. 1999; 13(2):115-20.

(77) Plato G. Der Weg zur Chronifizierung der kraniomandibulären Dysfunktionen (CMD). Manuelle Medizin. 2008; 46(6):384-5.

(78) Rocabado M. Diagnose und Behandlung einer abnormen kraniozervikalen und kraniomandibulären Mechanik. In: Solberg W, Clark G [Hrsg]. Kieferfunktion, Diagnostik und Therapie. 1. Auflage. Berlin: Quintessenz. 1985.

(79) Hülse M, Losert-Bruggner B. Der Einfluss der Kopfgelenke und/oder der Kiefergelenke auf die Hüftabduktion. Manuelle Medizin. 2002; 40(2):97-100.

(80) Deregibus A, Bracco P, Castroflorio T. Electromyographic analysis of masticatory and head and neck muscles related to therapy with functional appliances. Jahrbuch. ICCMO. 2003.

(81) Schupp W. Schmerz und Kieferorthopädie. Manuelle Medizin. 2000; 38(6): 322-8.

(82) Schupp W, Boissereé W, Haubrich J, Heller R, Marx G, Annunciato N, et al. Interdisciplinary cooperation between dentistry and manual medicine. The dentist's perspective. Manuelle Medizin. 2010; 48(3):192-8.

(83) Beyer L. Das tonische motorische System als Zielorgan manueller Behandlungstechniken. Manuelle Medizin. 2009; 47(2):99-106.

(84) Obata S, Kinoshita H. Chin force in violin playing. Eur J Appl Physiol. 2012; 112(6):2085-95.

(85) Philipson L, Sörbye R, Larsson P, Kaladjev S. Muscular load levels in performing musicians as monitored by quantitative electromyography. Med Probl Perform Art. 1990; 5:79-82.

(86) Dawson WJ, Charness M, Goode DJ, Lederman RJ, Newmark J. What's in a name? - Terminologic issues in performing arts medicine. Med Probl Perform Art. 1998; 13(2):45-50.

(87) Meinke WB. Risks and realities of musical performance. Med Probl Perform Art. 1998; 13:56-60.

(88) Nagai L, Eng J. Overuse injuries incurred by musicians. Physiotherapy Canada. 1992; 44:23-30.

(89) Kelleher LK, Campbell KR, Dickey JP. Biomechanical Research on Bowed String Musicians - A Scoping Study. Med Probl Perform Art. 2013; 28(4):212-8.

(90) Herman E. Orthodontic aspects of musical instrument selection. Am J Orthod. 1974; 65(5):519-30.

(91) Kovero O. Degenerative temporomandibular joint disease in a young violinist. Dentomaxillofac Radiol. 1989; 18(3):133-5.

(92)   Champagne D. Vann chin-rest. The Strad. 1979; 89:877-81.

(93)   Norris R. Applied ergonomics: adaptive equipment and instrument modification for musicians. Maryland medical journal. 1993; 42(3):271-5.

(94)   Scharf S. Muskuläre Inkoordination beim Musiker. Musikphysiologie und Musikermedizin. 1996; 3:82-8.

(95)   Järvholm U, Palmerud G, Styf J. Intramuscular pressure in the supraspinatus muscle. J Orthop Res. 1988; 6(2):230-8.

(96)   Järvholm U, Styf J, Suurkala M. Intramuscular pressure and muscle blood flow in supraspinatus. Eur J Appl Physiol. 1988; 58(3):219-24.

(97)   Järvholm U, Palmerud G, Herberts P. Intramuscular pressure and electromyography in the supraspinatus muscle at shoulder abduction. Clin Orthop Relat Res. 1989; 245:102-9.

(98)   Palmerud G, Forsman M, Sporrong H. Intramuscular pressure of the infra- and supraspinatus muscles in relation to hand load and arm posture. Eur J Appl Physiol. 2000; 83(2-3):223-30.

(99)   Wigaeus Tornqvist E, Kindenberg U, Schaerström A. Working Life Research in Europe. Stockholm: National Institute for Working Life. 2002; Report No 2:2002.

(100) Voight ML, Thomson BC. The role of the scapula in the rehabilitation of shoulder injuries. J Athl Train. 2000; 35(3):364-72.

(101) Paull B, Harrison C. The Athletic Musician: A Guide to Playing Without Pain. 1. Edition. Maryland: Scarecrow Press. 1997.

(102) Morin GE, Tiberio D, Austin G. The effect of upper trapezius taping on electro-myographic activity in the upper and middle trapezius region. Journal of Sports Rehabilitation. 1997; 6(4):309-18.

(103) Steinmetz A, Claus A, Hodges PW, Jull GA. Neck muscle function in violinists/ violists with and without neck pain. Clin Rheumatol. 2016; 35(4):1045-51.

(104) Cueco RT, Costa MG, Moral OM. Miofascial pain syndrome in young violin players [Presentation]. Sixth world congress on myofascial pain and fibromyalgia. Munich, 18.-22.07.2004.

(105) Kovero O, Könönen M, Pirinen S. The effect of violin playing on the bony facial structures in adolescents. Eur J Orthod. 1997; 19(4):369-75.

(106) Kiliaridis S. Masticatory muscle influence on craniofacial growth. Acta Odontol Scand. 1995; 53(3):196-202.

(107) O'Shaughnessy T. Craniomandibular/temporomandibular/cervical implications of a forced hyper-extension/hyper-flexion episode (i.e., whiplash). Funct Orthod. 1994; 11(2):5-12.

(108) Clemente M, Coimbra D, Silva A, Gabriel J, Aguiar Branco C, Pinho JC. Application of Infrared Thermal Imaging in a Violinist with Temporomandibular Disorder. Med Probl Perform Art. 2015; 30(4):251-4.

(109) Chojnowski M. Infrared thermal imaging in connective tissue diseases. Reumato-logia. 2017; 55(1):38-43.

(110) Clark GT, Green EM, Dornan MR, Flack VF. Craniocervical dysfunction levels in a patient sample from a temporomandibular joint clinic. J Am Dent Assoc. 1987; 115(2):251-6.

(111) Seedorf H, Toussaint R, Jakstat HA. Zusammenhänge zwischen Wirbelsäulen-Funktion, Beckentiefstand und kraniomandibulärer Dysfunktion. Dtsch Zahnarztl Z. 1999; 54:1-4.

(112) Kondo E, Aoba TJ. Case report of malocclusion with abnormal head posture and TMJ symptoms. Am J Orthod Dentofacial Orthop. 1999; 116(5):481-93.

(113) Lippold C. Beziehungen zwischen physiotherapeutischen und kieferorthopädischen Befunden. [Dissertation]. Münster: Medizinische Fakultät der Westfälischen Willhelms-Universität. 1999.

(114) Slavicek R. Funktion – die Haltung. In: Slavicek R [Hrsg]. Das Kauorgan: Funktionen und Dysfunktionen. 1. Auflage. Klosterneuburg: Gamma Medizinisch-wissenschaftliche Fortbildung. 2000.

(115) Kopp S, Seebald WG, Plato G. Kraniomandibuläre Dysfunktion – Eine Standortbestimmung. Manuelle Medizin. 2000; 38(6):335-41.

(116) Kopp S, Seebald WG, Plato G. Erkennen und Bewerten von Dysfunktionen und Schmerzphänomenen im kraniomandibulären System. Manuelle Medizin. 2000; 38(6):329-34.

(117) Danner HW, Jakstat HA, Ahlers MO. Correlations between posture and jaw relations. Z Kraniomandib Funkt. 2009; 1(2):149-63.

(118) Marx G. Über die Zusammenarbeit mit der Kieferorthopädie und Zahnheilkunde in der manuellen Medizin. Manuelle Medizin. 2000; 38(6):342-5.

(119) Schupp W, Haubrich J, Boisserée W, Läkamp M, Schuppan K. Interdisciplinary treatment of patients with craniomandibular dysfunctions. Manuelle Medizin. 2008; 46(6):393-400.

(120) Dworkin S. The case for incorporating biobehavioral treatment into TMD management. J Am Dent Assoc. 1996; 127(11):1607-10.

(121) Shargill I, Davie S, Al-ani Z. Treatment of temporomandibular disorder in a viola player—a case report. Dent Update. 2007; 34(3):181-4.

(122) Ferrario VF, Sforza C, Serrao G. The influence of crossbite on the coordinated electromyographic activity of human masticatory muscles during mastication. J Oral Rehabil. 1999; 26(7):575-81.

(123) Ferrario VF, Sforza C, Dellavia C, Tartaglia GM. Evidence of an influence of asymmetrical occlusal interferences on the activity of the sternocleidomastoid muscle. J Oral Rehabil. 2003; 30(1):34-40.

(124) Methfessel G. Funktionelle Prophylaxe bei Bläsern und Streichern. Jahrbuch der Hochschule für Musik Dresden. 2006. S. 102-107.

(125) Köneke C. Tinnitusbehandlung mit CMD-Therapie. ZWP 2004; 10(10):82-6.

(126) Peroz I. Tinnitus und Otalgien bei Funktionsstörungen des Kauorganes. In: Ahlers MO, Jakstat HA [Hrsg]. Klinische Funktionsanalyse. 3. Auflage. Hamburg: dentaConcept Verlag. 2007. S. 479-498.

(127) Kopp S, Friedrichs A, Pfaff G, Langbein U. Beeinflussung des funktionellen Bewegungsraumes von Hals-, Brust- und Lendenwirbelsäule durch Aufbissbehelfe. Eine Pilotstudie. Manuelle Medizin. 2003; 41(1):39-51.

(128) Toledo SD, Nadler SF, Norris RN, Akuthota V, Drake DF, Chou LH. Sports and performing arts medicine. 5. Issues relating to musicians. Arch Phys Med Rehabil. 2004; 85(3):72-4.

(129) Blum J, Ritter G. Violinists and violists with masses under the left side angle of the jaw known as 'fiddler's neck'. Med Probl Perform Art. 1990; 5(1):155-60.

(130) Brandfonbrener AG. Interview with Cho-Liang (Jimmy) Lin. Med Probl Perform Art. 1989; 4:3-8.

(131) Rabuffetti M, Converti R, Boccardi S, Ferrarin M. Tuning of the violin-performer interface: an experimental study about the effects of shoulder rest variations on playing kinematics. Med Probl Perform Art. 2007; 22(2):58-66.

(132) Harvell J, Maibach HI. Skin disease among musicians. Med Probl Perform Art. 1992; 7:114-20.

(133) Spahn C, Wasmer C, Eickhoff F, Nusseck M. Comparing violinists' body movements while standing, sitting, and in sitting orientations to the right or left of a music stand. Med Probl Perform Art. 2014; 29(2):86-93.

(134) Wright EF, Domenech MA, Fischer JR. Usefulness of posture training for patients with temporomandibular disorders. J Am Dent Assoc. 2000; 131(2):202-10.

(135) Berque P, Gray H. The influence of neck-shoulder pain on trapezius muscle activity among professional violin and viola players: an electromyographic study. Med Probl Perform Art. 2002; 17(2):68-75.

(136) Korbmacher H, Eggers-Stroeder G, Koch L, Kahl- Nieke B. Correlations between dentition anomalies and diseases of the postural and movement apparatus – a literature review. J Orofac Orthop. 2004; 65(3):190-203.

(137) Kopp S, Plato G, Sebald W. Interdisziplinäres Management von Patienten mit chronischem Schmerz. Z Bay. 1999; 10:6-10.

(138) Foxman I, Burgel BJ. Musician health and safety: Preventing playing-related musculoskeletal disorders. AAOHN J. 2006; 54(7):309-16.

(139) Lederman RJ. Neuromuscular and musculoskeletal problems in instrumental musicians. Muscle Nerve. 2003; 27(5):549-61.

(140) Ostwald PF, Baron BC, Byl NM, Wilson FR. Performing arts medicine. West J Med. 1994; 160(1):48-52.

(141) Ward MR. Myofascial pain in a young violin player: a case report. N Z Dent J. 1990; 86(386):92-3.

(142) de Souza Moraes GF, Antunes AP. Musculoskeletal disorders in professional violinists and violists. Systematic review. Acta Ortop Bras. 2012; 20(1):43-7.

(143) Atallah MM, Visscher CM, van Selms MKA, Lobbezoo F. Is there an association between temporomandibular disorders and playing a musical instrument? A review of literature. J Oral Rehabil. 2014; 41(7):532-41.

(144) van Selms MKA, Ahlberg J, Lobbezoo F, Visscher CM. Evidence-based review on temporomandibular disorders among musicians. Occup Med. 2017; 67(5):336-43.

Printed in the United States
By Bookmasters